the Complete CANINE HEALTH RECORD Book

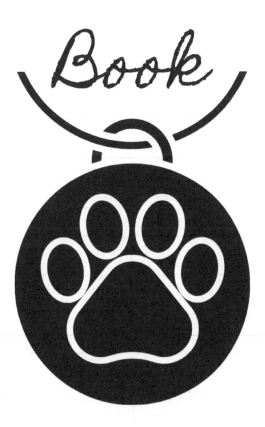

Canine Health Record © 2021 Sosha Publishing

CANINE INFORMATION

NAME:

BIRTHDATE: GENDER:

BREED: SPAYED/NEUTERED:

COAT COLOR: EYE COLOR:

MARKINGS:

OWNER(S):

ADDRESS:

PHONE: CELL:

E-MAIL:

BREEDER/SHELTER:

DATE ACQUIRED: REGISTERED NAME:

SIRE: DAM:

AKC #   REGISTRATION TYPE:

OTHER REGISTRY #   DNA #

MICROCHIP #   COMPANY:

VETERINARIAN:

EMERGENCY VET:

CANINE INFORMATION

WEIGHT	DATE	MEDICAL HISTORY
8 WEEKS:		
12 WEEKS:		
16 WEEKS:		
20 WEEKS:		
6 MONTHS:		
1 YEAR:		
2 YEARS:		
3 YEARS:		
4 YEARS:		
5 YEARS:		
6 YEARS:		
7 YEARS:		
8 YEARS:		
9 YEARS:		
10 YEARS:		
11 YEARS:		
12 YEARS:		
13 YEARS:		
14 YEARS:		

CANINE INFORMATION

WEIGHT		DATE	MEDICAL HISTORY
15 YEARS:			
16 YEARS:			
17 YEARS:			
18 YEARS:			
19 YEARS:			
20 YEARS:			
TRAINING CLASSES			

VACCINATIONS

VACCINE	DATES					NOTE
RABIES						
BORDATELLA						
LYNE DISEASE						
CORONAVIRUS						
PARVOVIRUS						
DISTEMPER						
PARAINFLUENZA						
LEPTOSPIROSIS						
CANINE INFLUENZA						
HEPATITIS/ADNOVIRUS						

OTHER TREATMENTS

HEARTWORM						
FLEA & TICK						

VACCINATIONS

VACCINE	DATES					NOTE
RABIES						
BORDATELLA						
LYNE DISEASE						
CORONAVIRUS						
PARVOVIRUS						
DISTEMPER						
PARAINFLUENZA						
LEPTOSPIROSIS						
CANINE INFLUENZA						
HEPATITIS/ADNOVIRUS						

OTHER TREATMENTS

HEARTWORM						
FLEA & TICK						

VACCINATIONS

VACCINE	DATES					NOTE
RABIES						
BORDATELLA						
LYNE DISEASE						
CORONAVIRUS						
PARVOVIRUS						
DISTEMPER						
PARAINFLUENZA						
LEPTOSPIROSIS						
CANINE INFLUENZA						
HEPATITIS/ADNOVIRUS						

OTHER TREATMENTS

HEARTWORM						
FLEA & TICK						

VACCINATIONS

VACCINE	DATES					NOTE
RABIES						
BORDATELLA						
LYNE DISEASE						
CORONAVIRUS						
PARVOVIRUS						
DISTEMPER						
PARAINFLUENZA						
LEPTOSPIROSIS						
CANINE INFLUENZA						
HEPATITIS/ADNOVIRUS						

OTHER TREATMENTS

HEARTWORM						
FLEA & TICK						

VACCINATIONS

VACCINE	DATES					NOTE
RABIES						
BORDATELLA						
LYNE DISEASE						
CORONAVIRUS						
PARVOVIRUS						
DISTEMPER						
PARAINFLUENZA						
LEPTOSPIROSIS						
CANINE INFLUENZA						
HEPATITIS/ADNOVIRUS						

OTHER TREATMENTS

HEARTWORM						
FLEA & TICK						

VET VISITATION LOG

DATE:	TIME:	VETERINARIAN:
April 8, 2024		

REASON FOR VISIT:

PHYSICAL — WNL

NEUROLOGICAL — NEEDS TO BE.... WNL

VACCINATIONS — CAN BE GIVEN

GROOMING — NEEDS A BATH AND NAILS EVERY OCCASION

NUTRITION — LID DUCK + HAIRCUT AND POTATO (1/4 CUP TWICE DAILY)

TREATMENT PLAN: TREATS SOMETIMES ONLY: TUDRA ORIJEN FLAVOR DUCK CRICKET TREATS JIMINY'S

TRAINING — CAN BE COMPLETED   KEEP CHECKING (FOR A-SHOTS)

— CAN CHECK IF HE REQUIRES ALLERGY SHOTS FOR MORE FOODS

— DENTAL CLEANING FOR DOGS OVER 2 (YEARLY)

— HAS TINY CAVITIES, CHECK WITH VET AND CONT BRUSHING

MEDICATIONS:

VACCINATIONS:

VISIT NOTES

VET VISITATION LOG

DATE: April 12, 2024   **TIME:** 9:05 AM   **VETERINARIAN:** Behavior + Social Skills + House Socialization—

REASON FOR VISIT: His training is not going well. He had exposure to a couple of dogs & hasn't responded. Play with them x. He is currently two years and four months old. Has not played with large / small dogs since two months old. Trauma born to eight weeks due to tail broken.

TREATMENT PLAN: Tues and Fri exposure — 8 month Puppy
An hr; May 5 to 6 hours necessary??
Will take notes.   4/16, 4/19, 4/23, 4/26
4/30, 5/3, 5/7, 5/10
5/14, 5/17, 5/21, 5/24

MEDICATIONS:

VACCINATIONS:

VISIT NOTES Training should be completed. He can buy new items the house will calm him without the colors. He is getting exposure therapy to dogs (trying to) until he joins the Shellby Semel trainings.

VET VISITATION LOG

DATE:	TIME:	VETERINARIAN:

REASON FOR VISIT:

TREATMENT PLAN:

MEDICATIONS:

VACCINATIONS:

VISIT NOTES

VET VISITATION LOG

DATE:	TIME:	VETERINARIAN:

REASON FOR VISIT:

_____

_____

_____

_____

TREATMENT PLAN:

_____

_____

_____

_____

MEDICATIONS:

_____

VACCINATIONS:

_____

VISIT NOTES

_____

_____

_____

_____

_____

VET VISITATION LOG

DATE:	TIME:	VETERINARIAN:

REASON FOR VISIT:

TREATMENT PLAN:

MEDICATIONS:

VACCINATIONS:

VISIT NOTES

VET VISITATION LOG

DATE:	TIME:	VETERINARIAN:

REASON FOR VISIT:

_____

_____

_____

_____

TREATMENT PLAN:

_____

_____

_____

_____

MEDICATIONS:

_____

VACCINATIONS:

_____

VISIT NOTES

_____

_____

_____

_____

_____

VET VISITATION LOG

DATE:	TIME:	VETERINARIAN:

REASON FOR VISIT:

TREATMENT PLAN:

MEDICATIONS:

VACCINATIONS:

VISIT NOTES

VET VISITATION LOG

DATE:	TIME:	VETERINARIAN:

REASON FOR VISIT:

_____

_____

_____

_____

_____

TREATMENT PLAN:

_____

_____

_____

_____

_____

MEDICATIONS:

_____

VACCINATIONS:

_____

_____

VISIT NOTES

_____

_____

_____

_____

_____

_____

VET VISITATION LOG

DATE:	TIME:	VETERINARIAN:

REASON FOR VISIT:

TREATMENT PLAN:

MEDICATIONS:

VACCINATIONS:

VISIT NOTES

VET VISITATION LOG

DATE:	TIME:	VETERINARIAN:

REASON FOR VISIT:

_____

_____

_____

_____

TREATMENT PLAN:

_____

_____

_____

_____

MEDICATIONS:

_____

VACCINATIONS:

_____

VISIT NOTES

_____

_____

_____

_____

_____

VET VISITATION LOG

DATE:	TIME:	VETERINARIAN:

REASON FOR VISIT:

_____

_____

_____

_____

_____

TREATMENT PLAN:

_____

_____

_____

_____

_____

MEDICATIONS:

_____

VACCINATIONS:

_____

VISIT NOTES

_____

_____

_____

_____

_____

_____

VET VISITATION LOG

DATE:	TIME:	VETERINARIAN:

REASON FOR VISIT:

_____

_____

_____

_____

TREATMENT PLAN:

_____

_____

_____

_____

MEDICATIONS:

_____

VACCINATIONS:

_____

VISIT NOTES

_____

_____

_____

_____

_____

VET VISITATION LOG

DATE:	TIME:	VETERINARIAN:

REASON FOR VISIT:

_____

_____

_____

_____

_____

TREATMENT PLAN:

_____

_____

_____

_____

_____

MEDICATIONS:

_____

VACCINATIONS:

_____

_____

VISIT NOTES

_____

_____

_____

_____

_____

_____

VET VISITATION LOG

DATE:	TIME:	VETERINARIAN:

REASON FOR VISIT:

TREATMENT PLAN:

MEDICATIONS:

VACCINATIONS:

VISIT NOTES

VET VISITATION LOG

DATE:	TIME:	VETERINARIAN:

REASON FOR VISIT:

_____

_____

_____

_____

_____

TREATMENT PLAN:

_____

_____

_____

_____

_____

MEDICATIONS:

VACCINATIONS:

_____

_____

VISIT NOTES

_____

_____

_____

_____

_____

_____

VET VISITATION LOG

DATE:	TIME:	VETERINARIAN:

REASON FOR VISIT:

_____

_____

_____

_____

_____

TREATMENT PLAN:

_____

_____

_____

_____

_____

MEDICATIONS:

_____

VACCINATIONS:

_____

_____

VISIT NOTES

_____

_____

_____

_____

_____

_____

VET VISITATION LOG

DATE:	TIME:	VETERINARIAN:

REASON FOR VISIT:

_____

_____

_____

_____

_____

TREATMENT PLAN:

_____

_____

_____

_____

_____

MEDICATIONS:

_____

VACCINATIONS:

_____

_____

VISIT NOTES

_____

_____

_____

_____

_____

VET VISITATION LOG

DATE:	TIME:	VETERINARIAN:

REASON FOR VISIT:

TREATMENT PLAN:

MEDICATIONS:

VACCINATIONS:

VISIT NOTES

VET VISITATION LOG

DATE:	TIME:	VETERINARIAN:

REASON FOR VISIT:

_____

_____

_____

_____

TREATMENT PLAN:

_____

_____

_____

_____

MEDICATIONS:

_____

VACCINATIONS:

_____

_____

VISIT NOTES

_____

_____

_____

_____

_____

VET VISITATION LOG

DATE:	TIME:	VETERINARIAN:

REASON FOR VISIT:

_____

_____

_____

_____

_____

TREATMENT PLAN:

_____

_____

_____

_____

_____

MEDICATIONS:

_____

VACCINATIONS:

_____

_____

VISIT NOTES

_____

_____

_____

_____

_____

_____

VET VISITATION LOG

DATE:	TIME:	VETERINARIAN:

REASON FOR VISIT:

TREATMENT PLAN:

MEDICATIONS:

VACCINATIONS:

VISIT NOTES

VET VISITATION LOG

DATE:	TIME:	VETERINARIAN:

REASON FOR VISIT:

_____

_____

_____

_____

_____

TREATMENT PLAN:

_____

_____

_____

_____

_____

MEDICATIONS:

_____

VACCINATIONS:

_____

VISIT NOTES

_____

_____

_____

_____

_____

_____

VET VISITATION LOG

DATE:	TIME:	VETERINARIAN:

REASON FOR VISIT:

_____

_____

_____

_____

_____

TREATMENT PLAN:

_____

_____

_____

_____

_____

MEDICATIONS:

_____

VACCINATIONS:

_____

_____

VISIT NOTES

_____

_____

_____

_____

_____

_____

VET VISITATION LOG

DATE:	TIME:	VETERINARIAN:

REASON FOR VISIT:

TREATMENT PLAN:

MEDICATIONS:

VACCINATIONS:

VISIT NOTES

VET VISITATION LOG

DATE:	TIME:	VETERINARIAN:

REASON FOR VISIT:

TREATMENT PLAN:

MEDICATIONS:

VACCINATIONS:

VISIT NOTES

VET VISITATION LOG

DATE:	TIME:	VETERINARIAN:

REASON FOR VISIT:

_____

_____

_____

_____

TREATMENT PLAN:

_____

_____

_____

_____

MEDICATIONS:

_____

VACCINATIONS:

_____

VISIT NOTES

_____

_____

_____

_____

_____

VET VISITATION LOG

DATE:	TIME:	VETERINARIAN:

REASON FOR VISIT:

TREATMENT PLAN:

MEDICATIONS:

VACCINATIONS:

VISIT NOTES

VET VISITATION LOG

DATE:	TIME:	VETERINARIAN:

REASON FOR VISIT:

_____

_____

_____

_____

_____

TREATMENT PLAN:

_____

_____

_____

_____

_____

MEDICATIONS:

_____

VACCINATIONS:

_____

VISIT NOTES

_____

_____

_____

_____

_____

_____

VET VISITATION LOG

DATE:	TIME:	VETERINARIAN:

REASON FOR VISIT:

_____

_____

_____

_____

_____

TREATMENT PLAN:

_____

_____

_____

_____

_____

MEDICATIONS:

_____

VACCINATIONS:

_____

_____

VISIT NOTES

_____

_____

_____

_____

_____

VET VISITATION LOG

DATE:	TIME:	VETERINARIAN:

REASON FOR VISIT:

_____

_____

_____

_____

TREATMENT PLAN:

_____

_____

_____

_____

MEDICATIONS:

_____

VACCINATIONS:

_____

VISIT NOTES

_____

_____

_____

_____

_____

VET VISITATION LOG

DATE:	TIME:	VETERINARIAN:

REASON FOR VISIT:

TREATMENT PLAN:

MEDICATIONS:

VACCINATIONS:

VISIT NOTES

VET VISITATION LOG

DATE:	TIME:	VETERINARIAN:

REASON FOR VISIT:

TREATMENT PLAN:

MEDICATIONS:

VACCINATIONS:

VISIT NOTES

VET VISITATION LOG

DATE:	TIME:	VETERINARIAN:

REASON FOR VISIT:

TREATMENT PLAN:

MEDICATIONS:

VACCINATIONS:

VISIT NOTES

VET VISITATION LOG

DATE:	TIME:	VETERINARIAN:

REASON FOR VISIT:

TREATMENT PLAN:

MEDICATIONS:

VACCINATIONS:

VISIT NOTES

VET VISITATION LOG

DATE:	TIME:	VETERINARIAN:

REASON FOR VISIT:

_____

_____

_____

_____

_____

TREATMENT PLAN:

_____

_____

_____

_____

_____

MEDICATIONS:

_____

VACCINATIONS:

_____

_____

VISIT NOTES

_____

_____

_____

_____

_____

_____

VET VISITATION LOG

DATE:	TIME:	VETERINARIAN:

REASON FOR VISIT:

TREATMENT PLAN:

MEDICATIONS:

VACCINATIONS:

VISIT NOTES

VET VISITATION LOG

DATE:	TIME:	VETERINARIAN:

REASON FOR VISIT:

TREATMENT PLAN:

MEDICATIONS:

VACCINATIONS:

VISIT NOTES

VET VISITATION LOG

DATE:	TIME:	VETERINARIAN:

REASON FOR VISIT:

TREATMENT PLAN:

MEDICATIONS:

VACCINATIONS:

VISIT NOTES

VET VISITATION LOG

DATE:	TIME:	VETERINARIAN:

REASON FOR VISIT:

TREATMENT PLAN:

MEDICATIONS:

VACCINATIONS:

VISIT NOTES

VET VISITATION LOG

DATE:	TIME:	VETERINARIAN:

REASON FOR VISIT:

_____

_____

_____

_____

TREATMENT PLAN:

_____

_____

_____

_____

MEDICATIONS:

_____

VACCINATIONS:

_____

VISIT NOTES

_____

_____

_____

_____

_____

CANINE

#2

CANINE

#2

CANINE INFORMATION

NAME:

BIRTHDATE: | GENDER:

BREED: | SPAYED/NEUTERED:

COAT COLOR: | EYE COLOR:

MARKINGS:

OWNER(S):

ADDRESS:

PHONE: | CELL:

E-MAIL:

BREEDER/SHELTER:

DATE ACQUIRED: | REGISTERED NAME:

SIRE: | DAM:

AKC # | REGISTRATION TYPE:

OTHER REGISTRY # | DNA #

MICROCHIP # | COMPANY:

VETERINARIAN:

EMERGENCY VET:

CANINE INFORMATION

WEIGHT	DATE	MEDICAL HISTORY
8 WEEKS:		
12 WEEKS:		
16 WEEKS:		
20 WEEKS:		
6 MONTHS:		
1 YEAR:		
2 YEARS:		
3 YEARS:		
4 YEARS:		
5 YEARS:		
6 YEARS:		
7 YEARS:		
8 YEARS:		
9 YEARS:		
10 YEARS:		
11 YEARS:		
12 YEARS:		
13 YEARS:		
14 YEARS:		

CANINE INFORMATION

WEIGHT		DATE	MEDICAL HISTORY
15 YEARS:			
16 YEARS:			
17 YEARS:			
18 YEARS:			
19 YEARS:			
20 YEARS:			
TRAINING CLASSES			

VACCINATIONS

VACCINE	DATES					NOTE
RABIES						
BORDATELLA						
LYNE DISEASE						
CORONAVIRUS						
PARVOVIRUS						
DISTEMPER						
PARAINFLUENZA						
LEPTOSPIROSIS						
CANINE INFLUENZA						
HEPATITIS/ADNOVIRUS						

OTHER TREATMENTS

HEARTWORM						
FLEA & TICK						

VACCINATIONS

VACCINE	DATES					NOTE
RABIES						
BORDATELLA						
LYNE DISEASE						
CORONAVIRUS						
PARVOVIRUS						
DISTEMPER						
PARAINFLUENZA						
LEPTOSPIROSIS						
CANINE INFLUENZA						
HEPATITIS/ADNOVIRUS						

OTHER TREATMENTS

HEARTWORM						
FLEA & TICK						

VACCINATIONS

VACCINE	DATES					NOTE
RABIES						
BORDATELLA						
LYNE DISEASE						
CORONAVIRUS						
PARVOVIRUS						
DISTEMPER						
PARAINFLUENZA						
LEPTOSPIROSIS						
CANINE INFLUENZA						
HEPATITIS/ADNOVIRUS						

OTHER TREATMENTS

HEARTWORM						
FLEA & TICK						

VACCINATIONS

VACCINE	DATES					NOTE
RABIES						
BORDATELLA						
LYNE DISEASE						
CORONAVIRUS						
PARVOVIRUS						
DISTEMPER						
PARAINFLUENZA						
LEPTOSPIROSIS						
CANINE INFLUENZA						
HEPATITIS/ADNOVIRUS						

OTHER TREATMENTS

HEARTWORM						
FLEA & TICK						

VACCINATIONS

VACCINE	DATES					NOTE
RABIES						
BORDATELLA						
LYNE DISEASE						
CORONAVIRUS						
PARVOVIRUS						
DISTEMPER						
PARAINFLUENZA						
LEPTOSPIROSIS						
CANINE INFLUENZA						
HEPATITIS/ADNOVIRUS						

OTHER TREATMENTS

HEARTWORM						
FLEA & TICK						

VET VISITATION LOG

DATE:	TIME:	VETERINARIAN:

REASON FOR VISIT:

_____

_____

_____

_____

TREATMENT PLAN:

_____

_____

_____

_____

MEDICATIONS:

_____

VACCINATIONS:

_____

VISIT NOTES

_____

_____

_____

_____

_____

VET VISITATION LOG

DATE:	TIME:	VETERINARIAN:

REASON FOR VISIT:

_____

_____

_____

_____

_____

TREATMENT PLAN:

_____

_____

_____

_____

_____

MEDICATIONS:

_____

VACCINATIONS:

_____

VISIT NOTES

_____

_____

_____

_____

_____

_____

VET VISITATION LOG

DATE:	TIME:	VETERINARIAN:

REASON FOR VISIT:

_____

_____

_____

_____

TREATMENT PLAN:

_____

_____

_____

_____

_____

MEDICATIONS:

_____

VACCINATIONS:

_____

VISIT NOTES

_____

_____

_____

_____

_____

_____

VET VISITATION LOG

DATE:	TIME:	VETERINARIAN:

REASON FOR VISIT:

TREATMENT PLAN:

MEDICATIONS:

VACCINATIONS:

VISIT NOTES

VET VISITATION LOG

DATE:	TIME:	VETERINARIAN:

REASON FOR VISIT:

_____

_____

_____

_____

_____

TREATMENT PLAN:

_____

_____

_____

_____

_____

MEDICATIONS:

_____

VACCINATIONS:

_____

_____

VISIT NOTES

_____

_____

_____

_____

_____

_____

VET VISITATION LOG

DATE:	TIME:	VETERINARIAN:

REASON FOR VISIT:

TREATMENT PLAN:

MEDICATIONS:

VACCINATIONS:

VISIT NOTES

VET VISITATION LOG

DATE:	TIME:	VETERINARIAN:

REASON FOR VISIT:

TREATMENT PLAN:

MEDICATIONS:

VACCINATIONS:

VISIT NOTES

VET VISITATION LOG

DATE:	TIME:	VETERINARIAN:

REASON FOR VISIT:

_____

_____

_____

_____

TREATMENT PLAN:

_____

_____

_____

_____

MEDICATIONS:

VACCINATIONS:

_____

VISIT NOTES

_____

_____

_____

_____

_____

VET VISITATION LOG

DATE:	TIME:	VETERINARIAN:

REASON FOR VISIT:

TREATMENT PLAN:

MEDICATIONS:

VACCINATIONS:

VISIT NOTES

VET VISITATION LOG

DATE:	TIME:	VETERINARIAN:

REASON FOR VISIT:

TREATMENT PLAN:

MEDICATIONS:

VACCINATIONS:

VISIT NOTES

VET VISITATION LOG

DATE:	TIME:	VETERINARIAN:

REASON FOR VISIT:

_____

_____

_____

_____

TREATMENT PLAN:

_____

_____

_____

_____

MEDICATIONS:

_____

VACCINATIONS:

_____

VISIT NOTES

_____

_____

_____

_____

_____

VET VISITATION LOG

DATE:	TIME:	VETERINARIAN:

REASON FOR VISIT:

_____

_____

_____

_____

TREATMENT PLAN:

_____

_____

_____

_____

MEDICATIONS:

VACCINATIONS:

_____

VISIT NOTES

_____

_____

_____

_____

_____

VET VISITATION LOG

DATE:	TIME:	VETERINARIAN:

REASON FOR VISIT:

TREATMENT PLAN:

MEDICATIONS:

VACCINATIONS:

VISIT NOTES

VET VISITATION LOG

DATE:	TIME:	VETERINARIAN:

REASON FOR VISIT:

_____

_____

_____

_____

TREATMENT PLAN:

_____

_____

_____

_____

MEDICATIONS:

VACCINATIONS:

_____

_____

VISIT NOTES

_____

_____

_____

_____

_____

_____

VET VISITATION LOG

DATE:	TIME:	VETERINARIAN:

REASON FOR VISIT:

TREATMENT PLAN:

MEDICATIONS:

VACCINATIONS:

VISIT NOTES

VET VISITATION LOG

DATE:	TIME:	VETERINARIAN:

REASON FOR VISIT:

_____

_____

_____

_____

_____

TREATMENT PLAN:

_____

_____

_____

_____

_____

MEDICATIONS:

VACCINATIONS:

_____

VISIT NOTES

_____

_____

_____

_____

_____

VET VISITATION LOG

DATE:	TIME:	VETERINARIAN:

REASON FOR VISIT:

_____

_____

_____

_____

TREATMENT PLAN:

_____

_____

_____

_____

MEDICATIONS:

_____

VACCINATIONS:

_____

_____

VISIT NOTES

_____

_____

_____

_____

_____

_____

VET VISITATION LOG

DATE:	TIME:	VETERINARIAN:

REASON FOR VISIT:

TREATMENT PLAN:

MEDICATIONS:

VACCINATIONS:

VISIT NOTES

VET VISITATION LOG

DATE:	TIME:	VETERINARIAN:

REASON FOR VISIT:

TREATMENT PLAN:

MEDICATIONS:

VACCINATIONS:

VISIT NOTES

VET VISITATION LOG

DATE:	TIME:	VETERINARIAN:

REASON FOR VISIT:

TREATMENT PLAN:

MEDICATIONS:

VACCINATIONS:

VISIT NOTES

VET VISITATION LOG

DATE:	TIME:	VETERINARIAN:

REASON FOR VISIT:

_____

_____

_____

_____

TREATMENT PLAN:

_____

_____

_____

_____

MEDICATIONS:

_____

VACCINATIONS:

_____

_____

VISIT NOTES

_____

_____

_____

_____

_____

VET VISITATION LOG

DATE:	TIME:	VETERINARIAN:

REASON FOR VISIT:

_____

_____

_____

_____

TREATMENT PLAN:

_____

_____

_____

_____

MEDICATIONS:

_____

VACCINATIONS:

_____

_____

VISIT NOTES

_____

_____

_____

_____

_____

VET VISITATION LOG

DATE:	TIME:	VETERINARIAN:

REASON FOR VISIT:

_____

_____

_____

_____

_____

TREATMENT PLAN:

_____

_____

_____

_____

_____

MEDICATIONS:

_____

VACCINATIONS:

_____

_____

VISIT NOTES

_____

_____

_____

_____

_____

_____

VET VISITATION LOG

DATE:	TIME:	VETERINARIAN:

REASON FOR VISIT:

_____

_____

_____

_____

TREATMENT PLAN:

_____

_____

_____

_____

MEDICATIONS:

VACCINATIONS:

_____

_____

VISIT NOTES

_____

_____

_____

_____

_____

_____

VET VISITATION LOG

DATE:	TIME:	VETERINARIAN:

REASON FOR VISIT:

TREATMENT PLAN:

MEDICATIONS:

VACCINATIONS:

VISIT NOTES

VET VISITATION LOG

DATE:	TIME:	VETERINARIAN:

REASON FOR VISIT:

_____

_____

_____

_____

TREATMENT PLAN:

_____

_____

_____

_____

MEDICATIONS:

_____

VACCINATIONS:

_____

_____

VISIT NOTES

_____

_____

_____

_____

_____

VET VISITATION LOG

DATE:	TIME:	VETERINARIAN:

REASON FOR VISIT:

TREATMENT PLAN:

MEDICATIONS:

VACCINATIONS:

VISIT NOTES

VET VISITATION LOG

DATE:	TIME:	VETERINARIAN:

REASON FOR VISIT:

_____

_____

_____

_____

TREATMENT PLAN:

_____

_____

_____

_____

MEDICATIONS:

VACCINATIONS:

_____

_____

VISIT NOTES

_____

_____

_____

_____

_____

VET VISITATION LOG

DATE:	TIME:	VETERINARIAN:

REASON FOR VISIT:

_____

_____

_____

_____

TREATMENT PLAN:

_____

_____

_____

_____

MEDICATIONS:

VACCINATIONS:

_____

_____

VISIT NOTES

_____

_____

_____

_____

_____

_____

VET VISITATION LOG

DATE:	TIME:	VETERINARIAN:

REASON FOR VISIT:

TREATMENT PLAN:

MEDICATIONS:

VACCINATIONS:

VISIT NOTES

VET VISITATION LOG

DATE:	TIME:	VETERINARIAN:

REASON FOR VISIT:

_____

_____

_____

_____

TREATMENT PLAN:

_____

_____

_____

_____

_____

MEDICATIONS:

_____

VACCINATIONS:

_____

VISIT NOTES

_____

_____

_____

_____

_____

VET VISITATION LOG

DATE:	TIME:	VETERINARIAN:

REASON FOR VISIT:

_____

_____

_____

_____

_____

TREATMENT PLAN:

_____

_____

_____

_____

_____

MEDICATIONS:

_____

VACCINATIONS:

_____

_____

VISIT NOTES

_____

_____

_____

_____

_____

_____

VET VISITATION LOG

DATE:	TIME:	VETERINARIAN:

REASON FOR VISIT:

TREATMENT PLAN:

MEDICATIONS:

VACCINATIONS:

VISIT NOTES

VET VISITATION LOG

DATE:	TIME:	VETERINARIAN:

REASON FOR VISIT:

TREATMENT PLAN:

MEDICATIONS:

VACCINATIONS:

VISIT NOTES

VET VISITATION LOG

DATE:	TIME:	VETERINARIAN:

REASON FOR VISIT:

_____

_____

_____

_____

TREATMENT PLAN:

_____

_____

_____

_____

MEDICATIONS:

VACCINATIONS:

_____

VISIT NOTES

_____

_____

_____

_____

_____

VET VISITATION LOG

DATE:	TIME:	VETERINARIAN:

REASON FOR VISIT:

TREATMENT PLAN:

MEDICATIONS:

VACCINATIONS:

VISIT NOTES

VET VISITATION LOG

DATE:	TIME:	VETERINARIAN:

REASON FOR VISIT:

_____

_____

_____

_____

_____

TREATMENT PLAN:

_____

_____

_____

_____

_____

MEDICATIONS:

_____

VACCINATIONS:

_____

_____

VISIT NOTES

_____

_____

_____

_____

_____

_____

VET VISITATION LOG

DATE:	TIME:	VETERINARIAN:

REASON FOR VISIT:

_____

_____

_____

_____

TREATMENT PLAN:

_____

_____

_____

_____

MEDICATIONS:

VACCINATIONS:

_____

_____

VISIT NOTES

_____

_____

_____

_____

_____

_____

VET VISITATION LOG

DATE:	TIME:	VETERINARIAN:

REASON FOR VISIT:

TREATMENT PLAN:

MEDICATIONS:

VACCINATIONS:

VISIT NOTES

VET VISITATION LOG

DATE:	TIME:	VETERINARIAN:

REASON FOR VISIT:

TREATMENT PLAN:

MEDICATIONS:

VACCINATIONS:

VISIT NOTES

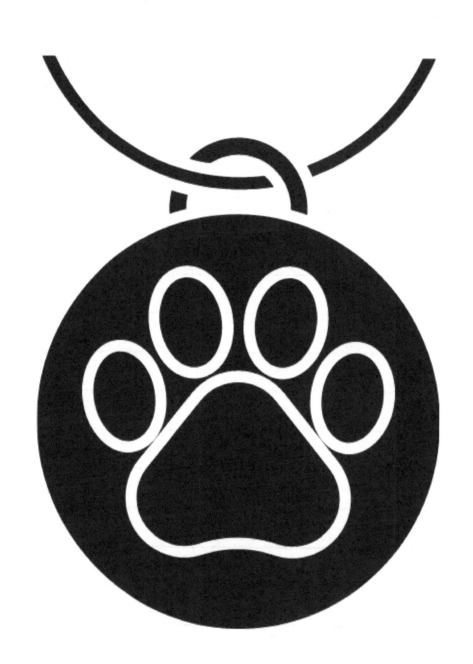

Made in United States
Troutdale, OR
04/02/2024